My Sauerkraut Log

Right Track Publishing

Olathe, KS

The Fervent Fermenter is *not* a series of How-To books. It is assumed that readers are relying on instructions and recipes from other sources. These journal-style logbooks are designed for keeping records of your forays into fermenting.
Happy adventures!

My Sauerkraut Log
The Fervent Fermenter Series
Published by Right Track Publishing in 2017
righttrackpublishing.com

The information provided in this publication is for educational and record-keeping purposes only, and is not intended to replace professional medical or nutritional advice.

ISBN: 978-0-9913371-7-0

Sauerkraut Basics

Sauerkraut is a special fermented dish made from finely shredded and salted cabbage. While many people think of it as a condiment to be used on hot dogs, polish sausage, and Reuben sandwiches, it also enjoyed as a side dish or snack.

Sauerkraut is an Eastern European tradition that has long been a part of Germanic cultures. It's rich in vitamins C and K, high in minerals calcium, potassium, and phosphorus, and high in probiotics. Sailors used to carry sauerkraut (sour cabbage) on voyages; it kept well and provided the necessary nutrients to prevent scurvy.

As any experienced home fermenter knows, raw sauerkraut made in one's own kitchen is nothing like the heat-treated, pasteurized and canned sauerkraut sitting on store shelves. It's filled with living enzymes and beneficial bacteria, and is high in antioxidants and dietary fiber.

The process of fermenting the cabbage in a brine solution is pretty straightforward, and there are several variations in addition to using cabbage only.

The final product and flavor will be a result of the temperature, length of fermentation, and the optional ingredients used to season it. That's why record-keeping is so helpful. Once you make a batch that's ooh-la-la, you will want to repeat your success over and over again.

For best results, it's recommended you follow the detailed directions from your favorite sauerkraut book or website. Always make sure your work area and equipment is sanitary.

You will need:

- ✔ Wide mouth mason jars or stoneware crock
- ✔ Utility knife or cabbage slicer
- ✔ Cutting board
- ✔ Large mixing bowl
- ✔ Airlock lids or crock lid

Ingredients:

- Cabbage (green, red, napa, or savoy)
- Kosher or sea salt
- Filtered water

Optional *(but probably not all at the same time): caraway seeds, juniper berries, red pepper flakes, coriander*

Sauerkraut can take anywhere from one to five weeks to ferment, depending on how thinly you slice the cabbage, how large the crock or vessel is, and the level of tartness you wish to achieve. Ideal room temperature is 60 to 72 degrees. When the sauerkraut is to your liking, refrigerate it.

You can make sauerkraut in glass canning jars or special stoneware pickling crocks with weighted stones to hold the cabbage down beneath the brine.

For instructions on making sauerkraut, please check out the following resources!

The resources below are great go-to's for beginners:

Websites

thekitchn.com/how-to-make-homemade-sauerkraut-in-a-mason-jar-193124

theprairiehomestead.com/2015/02/how-to-make-sauerkraut

culturesforhealth.com/learn/recipe/natural-fermentation/sauerkraut

toriavey.com/how-to/2013/06/how-to-ferment-cabbage-and-make-sauerkraut

Books

Ferment Your Vegetables: A Fun and Flavorful Guide to Making Your Own Pickles, Kimchi, Kraut, and More
by Amanda Feifer

Fermented Vegetables: Creative Recipes for Fermenting 64 Vegetables & Herbs in Krauts, Kimchis, Brined Pickles, Chutneys, Relishes & Pastes
by Christopher Shockey and Kirsten Shockey

Details

Vessel type and size ____________________

# of jars / crocks ________ Room Temp ______

Start Date ____________________

Cabbage type: ☐ green ☐ red

☐ napa ☐ savoy ☐ other

Additional ingredients: ____________________

____

____

☐ 1 week / flavor ____________________

☐ 2-week / flavor ____________________

☐ 3-week / flavor ____________________

☐ 4-week / flavor ____________________

Harvest Date: ____________________

Total # fermenting days _______

NOTES:

Details

Vessel type and size ____________________

# of jars / crocks ________ Room Temp ______

Start Date ____________________

Cabbage type: ☐ green ☐ red

☐ napa ☐ savoy ☐ other

Additional ingredients: ______________________

____

____

☐ 1 week / flavor _________________________

☐ 2-week / flavor _________________________

☐ 3-week / flavor _________________________

☐ 4-week / flavor _________________________

Harvest Date: ____________________

Total # fermenting days _______

NOTES:

Details

Vessel type and size ____________________

# of jars / crocks _______ Room Temp _____

Start Date ____________________

Cabbage type: ☐ green ☐ red

☐ napa ☐ savoy ☐ other

Additional ingredients: ____________________

____

____

☐ 1 week / flavor ____________________

☐ 2-week / flavor ____________________

☐ 3-week / flavor ____________________

☐ 4-week / flavor ____________________

Harvest Date: ____________________

Total # fermenting days ______

NOTES:

Details

Vessel type and size ____________________

# of jars / crocks ________ Room Temp ______

Start Date ____________________

Cabbage type: ☐ green ☐ red

☐ napa ☐ savoy ☐ other

Additional ingredients: ______________________
____
____

☐ 1 week / flavor __________________________

☐ 2-week / flavor __________________________

☐ 3-week / flavor __________________________

☐ 4-week / flavor __________________________

Harvest Date: ____________________

Total # fermenting days _______

NOTES:

Details

Vessel type and size ____________________

# of jars / crocks _______ Room Temp _____

Start Date ____________________

Cabbage type: ☐ green ☐ red

☐ napa ☐ savoy ☐ other

Additional ingredients: ____________________

____

____

☐ 1 week / flavor ____________________

☐ 2-week / flavor ____________________

☐ 3-week / flavor ____________________

☐ 4-week / flavor ____________________

Harvest Date: ____________________

Total # fermenting days ______

NOTES:

Details

Vessel type and size ____________________

# of jars / crocks ________ Room Temp ______

Start Date ____________________

Cabbage type: ☐ green ☐ red

☐ napa ☐ savoy ☐ other

Additional ingredients: ______________________
____
____

☐ 1 week / flavor ________________________

☐ 2-week / flavor ________________________

☐ 3-week / flavor ________________________

☐ 4-week / flavor ________________________

Harvest Date: ____________________

Total # fermenting days _______

NOTES:

DETAILS

Vessel type and size ______________________

# of jars / crocks ________ Room Temp ______

Start Date ______________________

Cabbage type: ☐ green ☐ red

☐ napa ☐ savoy ☐ other

Additional ingredients: ______________________

____

____

☐ 1 week / flavor ______________________

☐ 2-week / flavor ______________________

☐ 3-week / flavor ______________________

☐ 4-week / flavor ______________________

Harvest Date: ______________________

Total # fermenting days _______

NOTES:

Details

Vessel type and size ____________________

# of jars / crocks ________ Room Temp _____

Start Date ____________________

Cabbage type: ☐ green ☐ red

☐ napa ☐ savoy ☐ other

Additional ingredients: ____________________

____

____

☐ 1 week / flavor ____________________

☐ 2-week / flavor ____________________

☐ 3-week / flavor ____________________

☐ 4-week / flavor ____________________

Harvest Date: ____________________

Total # fermenting days ______

Notes:

Details

Vessel type and size ____________________

# of jars / crocks ________ Room Temp ______

Start Date ____________________

Cabbage type: ☐ green ☐ red

☐ napa ☐ savoy ☐ other

Additional ingredients: ______________________

____

____

☐ 1 week / flavor __________________________

☐ 2-week / flavor __________________________

☐ 3-week / flavor __________________________

☐ 4-week / flavor __________________________

Harvest Date: ____________________

Total # fermenting days _______

NOTES:

Details

Vessel type and size ______________________

# of jars / crocks ________ Room Temp ______

Start Date ______________________

Cabbage type: ☐ green ☐ red

☐ napa ☐ savoy ☐ other

Additional ingredients: ______________________

____

____

☐ 1 week / flavor ______________________

☐ 2-week / flavor ______________________

☐ 3-week / flavor ______________________

☐ 4-week / flavor ______________________

Harvest Date: ______________________

Total # fermenting days _______

NOTES:

Details

Vessel type and size ______________________

# of jars / crocks ________ Room Temp ______

Start Date ______________________

Cabbage type: ☐ green ☐ red

☐ napa ☐ savoy ☐ other

Additional ingredients: ______________________

____

____

☐ 1 week / flavor ______________________

☐ 2-week / flavor ______________________

☐ 3-week / flavor ______________________

☐ 4-week / flavor ______________________

Harvest Date: ______________________

Total # fermenting days _______

NOTES:

DETAILS

Vessel type and size ______________________

# of jars / crocks ________ Room Temp ______

Start Date ______________________

Cabbage type: ☐ green ☐ red

☐ napa ☐ savoy ☐ other

Additional ingredients: ______________________

____

____

☐ 1 week / flavor ______________________

☐ 2-week / flavor ______________________

☐ 3-week / flavor ______________________

☐ 4-week / flavor ______________________

Harvest Date: ______________________

Total # fermenting days ______

NOTES:

Details

Vessel type and size ____________________

# of jars / crocks ________ Room Temp ______

Start Date ____________________

Cabbage type: ☐ green ☐ red

☐ napa ☐ savoy ☐ other

Additional ingredients: ______________________

____

____

☐ 1 week / flavor _________________________

☐ 2-week / flavor _________________________

☐ 3-week / flavor _________________________

☐ 4-week / flavor _________________________

Harvest Date: ____________________

Total # fermenting days _______

NOTES:

Details

Vessel type and size ____________________

# of jars / crocks ________ Room Temp ______

Start Date ____________________

Cabbage type: ☐ green ☐ red

☐ napa ☐ savoy ☐ other

Additional ingredients: ______________________
____
____

☐ 1 week / flavor ______________________

☐ 2-week / flavor ______________________

☐ 3-week / flavor ______________________

☐ 4-week / flavor ______________________

Harvest Date: ____________________

Total # fermenting days _______

NOTES:

Details

Vessel type and size ____________________

# of jars / crocks ________ Room Temp ______

Start Date ____________________

Cabbage type: ☐ green ☐ red

☐ napa ☐ savoy ☐ other

Additional ingredients: ______________________

____

____

☐ 1 week / flavor __________________________

☐ 2-week / flavor __________________________

☐ 3-week / flavor __________________________

☐ 4-week / flavor __________________________

Harvest Date: ____________________

Total # fermenting days _______

NOTES:

Details

Vessel type and size ____________________

# of jars / crocks ________ Room Temp ______

Start Date ____________________

Cabbage type: ☐ green ☐ red

☐ napa ☐ savoy ☐ other

Additional ingredients: ______________________

____

____

☐ 1 week / flavor ________________________

☐ 2-week / flavor ________________________

☐ 3-week / flavor ________________________

☐ 4-week / flavor ________________________

Harvest Date: ____________________

Total # fermenting days _______

NOTES:

DETAILS

Vessel type and size ______________________

# of jars / crocks ________ Room Temp ______

Start Date ______________________

Cabbage type: ☐ green ☐ red

☐ napa ☐ savoy ☐ other

Additional ingredients: ______________________

____

____

☐ 1 week / flavor ______________________

☐ 2-week / flavor ______________________

☐ 3-week / flavor ______________________

☐ 4-week / flavor ______________________

Harvest Date: ______________________

Total # fermenting days _______

NOTES:

Details

Vessel type and size ____________________

# of jars / crocks ________ Room Temp ______

Start Date ____________________

Cabbage type: ☐ green ☐ red

☐ napa ☐ savoy ☐ other

Additional ingredients: ____________________

____

____

☐ 1 week / flavor ____________________

☐ 2-week / flavor ____________________

☐ 3-week / flavor ____________________

☐ 4-week / flavor ____________________

Harvest Date: ____________________

Total # fermenting days _______

NOTES:

DETAILS

Vessel type and size ______________________

# of jars / crocks ________ Room Temp _____

Start Date ______________________

Cabbage type: ☐ green ☐ red

☐ napa ☐ savoy ☐ other

Additional ingredients: ______________________

____

____

☐ 1 week / flavor __________________________

☐ 2-week / flavor __________________________

☐ 3-week / flavor __________________________

☐ 4-week / flavor __________________________

Harvest Date: ______________________

Total # fermenting days ______

NOTES:

DETAILS

Vessel type and size ______________________

# of jars / crocks ________ Room Temp ______

Start Date ______________________

Cabbage type: ☐ green ☐ red

☐ napa ☐ savoy ☐ other

Additional ingredients: ______________________

____

____

☐ 1 week / flavor ______________________

☐ 2-week / flavor ______________________

☐ 3-week / flavor ______________________

☐ 4-week / flavor ______________________

Harvest Date: ______________________

Total # fermenting days _______

NOTES:

Details

Vessel type and size ______________________

# of jars / crocks ________ Room Temp ______

Start Date ______________________

Cabbage type: ☐ green ☐ red

☐ napa ☐ savoy ☐ other

Additional ingredients: ______________________

____

____

☐ 1 week / flavor ______________________

☐ 2-week / flavor ______________________

☐ 3-week / flavor ______________________

☐ 4-week / flavor ______________________

Harvest Date: ______________________

Total # fermenting days _______

NOTES:

Details

Vessel type and size ____________________

# of jars / crocks ________ Room Temp ______

Start Date ____________________

Cabbage type: ☐ green ☐ red

☐ napa ☐ savoy ☐ other

Additional ingredients: ______________________

____

____

☐ 1 week / flavor __________________________

☐ 2-week / flavor __________________________

☐ 3-week / flavor __________________________

☐ 4-week / flavor __________________________

Harvest Date: ____________________

Total # fermenting days _______

NOTES:

Details

Vessel type and size ______________________

\# of jars / crocks ________ Room Temp ______

Start Date ______________________

Cabbage type: ☐ green ☐ red

☐ napa ☐ savoy ☐ other

Additional ingredients: ______________________

____

____

☐ 1 week / flavor ______________________

☐ 2-week / flavor ______________________

☐ 3-week / flavor ______________________

☐ 4-week / flavor ______________________

Harvest Date: ______________________

Total # fermenting days _______

NOTES:

DETAILS

Vessel type and size ______________________

# of jars / crocks ________ Room Temp _____

Start Date ______________________

Cabbage type: ☐ green ☐ red

☐ napa ☐ savoy ☐ other

Additional ingredients: ______________________

____

____

☐ 1 week / flavor ______________________

☐ 2-week / flavor ______________________

☐ 3-week / flavor ______________________

☐ 4-week / flavor ______________________

Harvest Date: ______________________

Total # fermenting days ______

NOTES:

Details

Vessel type and size ______________________

# of jars / crocks ________ Room Temp ______

Start Date ______________________

Cabbage type: ☐ green ☐ red

☐ napa ☐ savoy ☐ other

Additional ingredients: ______________________

____

____

☐ 1 week / flavor ______________________

☐ 2-week / flavor ______________________

☐ 3-week / flavor ______________________

☐ 4-week / flavor ______________________

Harvest Date: ______________________

Total # fermenting days _______

NOTES:

Details

Vessel type and size ________________

# of jars / crocks ________ Room Temp ______

Start Date ________________

Cabbage type: ☐ green ☐ red

☐ napa ☐ savoy ☐ other

Additional ingredients: ______________________

____

____

☐ 1 week / flavor ______________________

☐ 2-week / flavor ______________________

☐ 3-week / flavor ______________________

☐ 4-week / flavor ______________________

Harvest Date: ________________

Total # fermenting days _______

Notes:

Details

Vessel type and size ______________________

# of jars / crocks ________ Room Temp ______

Start Date ______________________

Cabbage type: ☐ green ☐ red

☐ napa ☐ savoy ☐ other

Additional ingredients: ______________________

____

____

☐ 1 week / flavor ______________________

☐ 2-week / flavor ______________________

☐ 3-week / flavor ______________________

☐ 4-week / flavor ______________________

Harvest Date: ______________________

Total # fermenting days _______

NOTES:

Details

Vessel type and size ____________________

# of jars / crocks ________ Room Temp ______

Start Date ____________________

Cabbage type: ☐ green ☐ red

☐ napa ☐ savoy ☐ other

Additional ingredients: ______________________

____

____

☐ 1 week / flavor ________________________

☐ 2-week / flavor ________________________

☐ 3-week / flavor ________________________

☐ 4-week / flavor ________________________

Harvest Date: ____________________

Total # fermenting days _______

NOTES:

Details

Vessel type and size ______________________

# of jars / crocks ________ Room Temp ______

Start Date ______________________

Cabbage type: ☐ green ☐ red

☐ napa ☐ savoy ☐ other

Additional ingredients: ______________________

____

____

☐ 1 week / flavor ______________________

☐ 2-week / flavor ______________________

☐ 3-week / flavor ______________________

☐ 4-week / flavor ______________________

Harvest Date: ______________________

Total # fermenting days _______

NOTES:

Details

Vessel type and size ______________________

# of jars / crocks ________ Room Temp ______

Start Date ______________________

Cabbage type: ☐ green ☐ red

☐ napa ☐ savoy ☐ other

Additional ingredients: ______________________

____

____

☐ 1 week / flavor ______________________

☐ 2-week / flavor ______________________

☐ 3-week / flavor ______________________

☐ 4-week / flavor ______________________

Harvest Date: ______________________

Total # fermenting days _______

Notes:

DETAILS

Vessel type and size ________________________

# of jars / crocks ________ Room Temp ______

Start Date ________________________

Cabbage type: ☐ green ☐ red

☐ napa ☐ savoy ☐ other

Additional ingredients: ________________________

____

____

☐ 1 week / flavor ________________________

☐ 2-week / flavor ________________________

☐ 3-week / flavor ________________________

☐ 4-week / flavor ________________________

Harvest Date: ________________________

Total # fermenting days _______

NOTES:

DETAILS

Vessel type and size ______________________

# of jars / crocks ________ Room Temp ______

Start Date ______________________

Cabbage type: ☐ green ☐ red

☐ napa ☐ savoy ☐ other

Additional ingredients: ______________________

____

____

☐ 1 week / flavor ______________________

☐ 2-week / flavor ______________________

☐ 3-week / flavor ______________________

☐ 4-week / flavor ______________________

Harvest Date: ______________________

Total # fermenting days _______

NOTES:

Details

Vessel type and size ____________________

# of jars / crocks ________ Room Temp ______

Start Date ____________________

Cabbage type: ☐ green ☐ red

☐ napa ☐ savoy ☐ other

Additional ingredients: ______________________

____

____

☐ 1 week / flavor ________________________

☐ 2-week / flavor ________________________

☐ 3-week / flavor ________________________

☐ 4-week / flavor ________________________

Harvest Date: ____________________

Total # fermenting days _______

NOTES:

Details

Vessel type and size ______________________

# of jars / crocks ________ Room Temp ______

Start Date ______________________

Cabbage type: ☐ green ☐ red

☐ napa ☐ savoy ☐ other

Additional ingredients: ______________________

____

____

☐ 1 week / flavor ______________________

☐ 2-week / flavor ______________________

☐ 3-week / flavor ______________________

☐ 4-week / flavor ______________________

Harvest Date: ______________________

Total # fermenting days ______

NOTES:

Details

Vessel type and size ______________________

# of jars / crocks ________ Room Temp ______

Start Date ______________________

Cabbage type: ☐ green ☐ red

☐ napa ☐ savoy ☐ other

Additional ingredients: ______________________

____

____

☐ 1 week / flavor ______________________

☐ 2-week / flavor ______________________

☐ 3-week / flavor ______________________

☐ 4-week / flavor ______________________

Harvest Date: ______________________

Total # fermenting days _______

Notes:

DETAILS

Vessel type and size ______________________

# of jars / crocks ________ Room Temp ______

Start Date ______________________

Cabbage type: ☐ green ☐ red

☐ napa ☐ savoy ☐ other

Additional ingredients: ______________________

____

____

☐ 1 week / flavor ______________________

☐ 2-week / flavor ______________________

☐ 3-week / flavor ______________________

☐ 4-week / flavor ______________________

Harvest Date: ______________________

Total # fermenting days _______

NOTES:

Details

Vessel type and size ______________________

# of jars / crocks ________ Room Temp ______

Start Date ______________________

Cabbage type: ☐ green ☐ red

☐ napa ☐ savoy ☐ other

Additional ingredients: ______________________

____

____

☐ 1 week / flavor ______________________

☐ 2-week / flavor ______________________

☐ 3-week / flavor ______________________

☐ 4-week / flavor ______________________

Harvest Date: ______________________

Total # fermenting days _______

NOTES:

Details

Vessel type and size ____________________

# of jars / crocks ________ Room Temp ______

Start Date ____________________

Cabbage type: ☐ green ☐ red

☐ napa ☐ savoy ☐ other

Additional ingredients: ____________________

____

____

☐ 1 week / flavor ____________________

☐ 2-week / flavor ____________________

☐ 3-week / flavor ____________________

☐ 4-week / flavor ____________________

Harvest Date: ____________________

Total # fermenting days _______

NOTES:

DETAILS

Vessel type and size ________________________

# of jars / crocks ________ Room Temp ______

Start Date ________________________

Cabbage type: ☐ green ☐ red

☐ napa ☐ savoy ☐ other

Additional ingredients: ______________________

____

____

☐ 1 week / flavor __________________________

☐ 2-week / flavor __________________________

☐ 3-week / flavor __________________________

☐ 4-week / flavor __________________________

Harvest Date: ________________________

Total # fermenting days _______

NOTES:

Details

Vessel type and size ______________________

# of jars / crocks ________ Room Temp ______

Start Date ______________________

Cabbage type: ☐ green ☐ red

☐ napa ☐ savoy ☐ other

Additional ingredients: ______________________

____

____

☐ 1 week / flavor ______________________

☐ 2-week / flavor ______________________

☐ 3-week / flavor ______________________

☐ 4-week / flavor ______________________

Harvest Date: ______________________

Total # fermenting days ______

NOTES:

DETAILS

Vessel type and size ____________________

# of jars / crocks ________ Room Temp ______

Start Date ____________________

Cabbage type: ☐ green ☐ red

☐ napa ☐ savoy ☐ other

Additional ingredients: ______________________

____

____

☐ 1 week / flavor ______________________

☐ 2-week / flavor ______________________

☐ 3-week / flavor ______________________

☐ 4-week / flavor ______________________

Harvest Date: ____________________

Total # fermenting days _______

NOTES:

Details

Vessel type and size ____________________

# of jars / crocks ________ Room Temp ______

Start Date ____________________

Cabbage type: ☐ green ☐ red

☐ napa ☐ savoy ☐ other

Additional ingredients: ______________________

____

____

☐ 1 week / flavor ______________________

☐ 2-week / flavor ______________________

☐ 3-week / flavor ______________________

☐ 4-week / flavor ______________________

Harvest Date: ____________________

Total # fermenting days _______

NOTES:

Details

Vessel type and size ____________________

# of jars / crocks ________ Room Temp ______

Start Date ____________________

Cabbage type: ☐ green ☐ red

☐ napa ☐ savoy ☐ other

Additional ingredients: ______________________

____

____

☐ 1 week / flavor _________________________

☐ 2-week / flavor _________________________

☐ 3-week / flavor _________________________

☐ 4-week / flavor _________________________

Harvest Date: ____________________

Total # fermenting days _______

NOTES:

DETAILS

Vessel type and size ________________

# of jars / crocks ________ Room Temp ______

Start Date ________________

Cabbage type: ☐ green ☐ red

☐ napa ☐ savoy ☐ other

Additional ingredients: ______________________

____

____

☐ 1 week / flavor ________________________

☐ 2-week / flavor ________________________

☐ 3-week / flavor ________________________

☐ 4-week / flavor ________________________

Harvest Date: ________________

Total # fermenting days _______

NOTES:

Details

Vessel type and size ______________________

# of jars / crocks ________ Room Temp ______

Start Date ______________________

Cabbage type: ☐ green ☐ red

☐ napa ☐ savoy ☐ other

Additional ingredients: ______________________

____

____

☐ 1 week / flavor ______________________

☐ 2-week / flavor ______________________

☐ 3-week / flavor ______________________

☐ 4-week / flavor ______________________

Harvest Date: ______________________

Total # fermenting days _______

NOTES:

DETAILS

Vessel type and size ______________________

# of jars / crocks ________ Room Temp ______

Start Date ______________________

Cabbage type: ☐ green ☐ red

☐ napa ☐ savoy ☐ other

Additional ingredients: ______________________

____

____

☐ 1 week / flavor ______________________

☐ 2-week / flavor ______________________

☐ 3-week / flavor ______________________

☐ 4-week / flavor ______________________

Harvest Date: ______________________

Total # fermenting days _______

NOTES:

DETAILS

Vessel type and size ______________________

# of jars / crocks ________ Room Temp ______

Start Date ______________________

Cabbage type: ☐ green ☐ red

☐ napa ☐ savoy ☐ other

Additional ingredients: ______________________

____

____

☐ 1 week / flavor ______________________

☐ 2-week / flavor ______________________

☐ 3-week / flavor ______________________

☐ 4-week / flavor ______________________

Harvest Date: ______________________

Total # fermenting days _______

NOTES:

Details

Vessel type and size ____________________

# of jars / crocks ________ Room Temp ______

Start Date ____________________

Cabbage type: ☐ green ☐ red

☐ napa ☐ savoy ☐ other

Additional ingredients: ______________________

____

____

☐ 1 week / flavor ________________________

☐ 2-week / flavor ________________________

☐ 3-week / flavor ________________________

☐ 4-week / flavor ________________________

Harvest Date: ____________________

Total # fermenting days _______

NOTES:

DETAILS

Vessel type and size ____________________

# of jars / crocks ________ Room Temp ______

Start Date ____________________

Cabbage type: ☐ green ☐ red

☐ napa ☐ savoy ☐ other

Additional ingredients: ______________________

____

____

☐ 1 week / flavor ________________________

☐ 2-week / flavor ________________________

☐ 3-week / flavor ________________________

☐ 4-week / flavor ________________________

Harvest Date: ____________________

Total # fermenting days _______

NOTES:

DETAILS

Vessel type and size ______________________

# of jars / crocks ________ Room Temp ______

Start Date ______________________

Cabbage type: ☐ green ☐ red

☐ napa ☐ savoy ☐ other

Additional ingredients: ______________________

____

____

☐ 1 week / flavor ______________________

☐ 2-week / flavor ______________________

☐ 3-week / flavor ______________________

☐ 4-week / flavor ______________________

Harvest Date: ______________________

Total # fermenting days _______

NOTES:

Made in the USA
Monee, IL
04 November 2026

67386076R10059